Copyright

All rights reserved. No part of this publication may be reproduced, distributed, or transmitted in any form or by any means, including photocopying, recording, or other electronic or mechanical methods, without the prior written permission of the publisher, except in the case of brief quotations embodied in critical reviews and certain other noncommercial uses permitted by copyright law

1

Table of Contents

INTRODUCTION

Pancreatitis is a disease in which your pancreas becomes inflamed. The pancreas is a large gland behind your stomach and next to your small intestine.

The pancreas does two main things:

1. It releases powerful digestive enzymes into your small intestine to help you digest food.
2. It releases insulin and glucagon into your bloodstream. These hormones help your body control how it uses food for energy.

The pancreas can have issues when digestive enzymes begin working before the pancreas releases them.

Pancreatitis Symptoms

Pancreatitis can suddenly manifest itself and can be diagnosed as either mild, acute, or chronic pancreatitis. Mild pancreatitis may heal on its own without treatment but if left unchecked can progress to severe and life-threatening complications.

The signs and symptoms of pancreatitis are not the same for each person. Mild to acute cases of pancreatitis can have the following symptoms :

- Fever
- Higher heart rate
- Nausea and vomiting
- Swollen and tender belly

- Pain in the upper part of your belly that goes into your back. Eating may make it worse, especially foods high in fat.

It is advised to consult your doctor immediately should you feel persistent pain in the abdomen and if the pain keeps you from comfortably sitting down.

Pancreatitis Complications

Pancreatitis can have severe complications, including:

1. Diabetes, if there's damage to the cells that produce insulin

2. Infection of your pancreas

3. Kidney failure

4. Malnutrition, if your body can't get enough nutrients from the food you eat because of a lack of digestive enzymes

5. Pancreatic cancer

6. Pancreatic necrosis, when tissues die because your pancreas isn't getting enough blood

7. Problems with your breathing when chemical changes in your body affect your lungs

8. Pseudocysts, when fluid collects in pockets on your pancreas. They can burst and become infected.

What to eat if you have pancreatitis

To get your pancreas healthy, focus on foods that are rich in protein, low in animal fats, and contain antioxidants. Try lean meats, beans and lentils, clear soups, and dairy alternatives (such as flax milk and almond milk). Your pancreas won't have to work as hard to process these.

Research suggests that some people with pancreatitis can tolerate up to 30 to 40% of calories from fat when it's from whole-food plant sources or medium-chain triglycerides (MCTs). Others do better with much lower fat intake, such as 50 grams or less per day.

Spinach, blueberries, cherries, and whole grains can work to protect your digestion and fight the free radicals that damage your organs.

If you're craving something sweet, reach for fruit instead of added sugars since those with pancreatitis are at high risk for diabetes.

Consider cherry tomatoes, cucumbers and hummus, and fruit as your go-to snacks. Your pancreas will thank you.

What not to eat if you have pancreatitis

Foods to limit include:

- red meat
- organ meats

- fried foods

- fries and potato chips

- mayonnaise

- margarine and butter

- full-fat dairy

- pastries and desserts with added sugars

- beverages with added sugars

- Avoid trans-fatty acids in your diet.

Fried or heavily processed foods, like french fries and fast-food hamburgers, are some of the worst offenders. Organ meats, full-fat dairy, potato chips, and mayonnaise also top the list of foods to limit.

Cooked or deep-fried foods might trigger a flare-up of pancreatitis. You'll also want to cut back on the refined flour found in cakes, pastries, and cookies. These foods can tax the digestive system by causing your insulin levels to spike.

NUTRITIONAL ADVICE & RECIPES

This is a very important section because the quality of life is important for all of us but is certainly much more of a challenge for individuals and their loved ones trying to manage chronic illness.

This book provides support and information on all aspects of daily life, including nutrition, and practical tips.

For patients with pancreatic disease, there are many times when it is difficult to eat at all. Even when you are feeling well, you still have to be very careful to follow a low-fat diet. Below are some guidelines, and, as always, your doctor is the best one to tell you how to eat. Note that sometimes it is easier to eat small meals several times a day, instead of trying to sit down to three big meals.

A low-fat diet

The amount of fat you should eat varies depending on your weight and height, but for an average person, it is felt that you should not consume more than 50 grams of fat a day. Fat intake could range between 30-50 grams of fat, depending on tolerance. Daily fat consumption should not be

14

concentrated in one meal but spread throughout the day in possibly 4-6 small meals. Eating boneless chicken breasts and most fish helps keep your meals low in fat. Cooking with Pam or any cooking spray instead of oils also helps. You can add fat-free chicken broth when you need moisture.

Alcohol and dehydration

If you have pancreatic disease, it is important to never drink alcohol. Research has shown that dehydration causes the pancreas to flare. Always drink plenty of fluid. It has been recommended that a patient always have a bottle of water or any liquid with them at all times. Drinking Gatorade or other sports drinks is a good way to keep from being dehydrated.

Taking a break

Sometimes it is best to rest the pancreas and limit your food intake. If you are experiencing a flare, your doctor may even recommend no food for a day or two. A diet of clear liquids can be followed when pain is severe. Clear liquids include apple, cranberry and white grape juice, gelatin and broth. The clear liquid diet, however, is not nutritionally complete and the diet should be advanced as soon as additional food is tolerated and according to the schedule given to you by your doctor.

MEAL RECIPES

1. APPLE BUTTERNUT SQUASH PANCAKES

These delicious pancakes can be used as a meal any time of the day. They are rich in beta-carotene and are designed to be easy to tolerate for pancreatic cancer symptoms such as nausea and overall stomach upset. For additional protein, nuts can be added. For those who are experiencing fat intolerance, reduced fat versions of the dairy components can be substituted, along with lower lactose alternatives for those with lactose intolerance.

For those on more severe fiber restrictions, the apple and squash components can also be

peeled and boiled to help break down some of the fibers for optimal digestive tolerance.

These can also be easily frozen (with layers of parchment paper in between) and reheated in the toaster oven or microwave.

Yield: 12 small pancakes (6 large)

INGREDIENTS:

- 3 cups grated raw butternut squash or acorn squash (may also use zucchini)
- 1 large green apple (or 2 small) grated, raw

- 1/3 cup sour cream (use reduced-fat or vegan sour cream if necessary)
- 1 egg
- 1/4 cup milk of choice (use lactose-free,
- non-dairy, or reduced-fat as needed)
- 1 cup all-purpose flour
- 1 tsp. baking powder
- 1 tsp. baking soda
- 1 tsp. cinnamon

DIRECTIONS:

1. Grate squash on cheese grater or food processor. Steam in a shallow bowl in microwave with a small amount of water for 3 minutes to soften.

2. Core and grate apple on cheese grater or food processor, and add to squash mixture.

3. Add squash and apple to a mixing bowl and stir in sour cream, egg, and milk with a fork.

4. In a separate bowl, sift flour, baking powder, baking soda, and cinnamon. Add to mixing bowl and stir with the fork.

5. Heat frying pan to low-medium and spray with cooking spray.

6. Using a ladle or a spoon, drop batter onto pan into small pancakes. Flip when bubbles start to form around the edges of pancake.

NUTRITIONAL DATA: 166 calories, 3.9 grams fat, 2.1 grams saturated fat, 34 mg cholesterol,

29.8 grams carbohydrate, 2.9 grams dietary fiber,

4.4 grams protein

2. PASTIERA (PASTA EGG BAKE)

Pastiera is traditionally an Italian-style Easter cake

that is sweetened and made with ricotta cheese.

This recipe is a savory spin on this classic dish and

is packed with protein from the eggs and milk.

Lactose-free milk and cheese can be used for those

experiencing lactose intolerance. Spaghetti squash

is also a great substitution for pasta noodles as a

lower carbohydrate alternative or for those looking

to add a tolerable vegetable component.

Yield: 8 servings

INGREDIENTS:

- 12 eggs, beaten (may substitute for lower fat pasteurized liquid egg product)
- 2 cups of milk (substitute non-fat or reduced fat milk if experiencing fat intolerance)
- Salt and pepper to taste
- 1 cup of grated Parmesan cheese
- Perciatelli (aka Bucatini or #6 macaroni spaghetti with a hole running through)

DIRECTIONS:

1. Preheat oven to 250°. Spray a rectangular 9x13" baking dish with nonfat cooking spray.

2. Cook pasta according to package directions.

3. Mix beaten eggs with milk, salt, pepper, and cheese while macaroni is cooking.

4. Combine together in the 9x13" baking dish.

5. Bake at 250° for 10 minutes, and then increase oven temperature to 350° for 25-30 minutes.

6. Cut into 8 pieces, or smaller as a side dish.

NUTRITIONAL DATA:

378 calories, 11.5 grams fat, 4.6 grams saturated fat, 259 mg cholesterol, 48.5 grams carbohydrate, 2 grams dietary fiber, 21.4 grams protein

3. THANKSGIVING MEATBALLS

This is a unique twist to a comfort food that takes meatballs from savory to slightly

sweet. It's a great choice for those needing low-fat protein choices during the holiday.

Yield: 16 medium sized meatballs, 8 servings

INGREDIENTS:

- 1 1/2 lb. ground turkey meat (you can use half ground turkey and half sweet turkey sausage for extra flavor)
- 1 1/4 cup of herbed stuffing bread cubes
- 1/2 cup dried cranberries
- 1 large egg plus 1 egg white

- 1/4 cup finely chopped sweet onion

- 1 Tbsp. chopped fresh sage

- 1 tsp. salt

- 1 Tbsp. olive oil

- Other add-in ideas: shredded carrots or chopped mushrooms

DIRECTIONS:

1. Preheat oven to 450°.

2. Coat a 9x13 inch baking sheet with olive oil and set aside.

3. In a large bowl, combine the ground turkey/turkey sausage, cranberries, eggs, onion, sage, and salt.

25

4. Add half of the stuffing cubes in whole form, and crush the other half in your hands to resemble bread crumbs. Mix everything together with your hands until it is all incorporated.

5. Coat your hands with a little bit of olive oil and roll the mixture firmly into balls about the size of golf balls.

6. Place the meatballs in the baking dish directly next to each other in rows. This will help them keep their shape while baking.

7. Roast for about 20 minutes, until the meatballs are cooked through and slightly brown on top.

8. Serve meatballs with gravy and cranberry sauce, and enjoy.

NUTRITIONAL DATA:

192 calories, 7.9 grams fat, 1.8 grams saturated fat, 73 mg cholesterol, 5.4 grams carbohydrate, 0.9 grams dietary fiber, 18.5 grams protein

4. MAPLE GREEN BEANS

Roasting green beans is a quick and easy way to prepare a delicious green vegetable.

This recipe can be made with fresh out-of-the-garden green beans, fresh packaged and pre-washed green beans, or frozen green beans. Boost the flavor by using pure maple syrup.

Yield: 4 Servings

INGREDIENTS:

- 1 lb. green beans
- 1 Tbsp. maple syrup
- 1 tsp. olive oil
- 1/2 tsp. salt
- 1/4 tsp. pepper

DIRECTIONS:

1. Preheat oven to 400°.
2. In a large bowl, toss green beans with maple syrup, oil, salt and pepper.
3. Arrange evenly on sheet tray.
4. Roast until tender, about 20 to 25 minutes.

NUTRITIONAL DATA:

59 calories, 1.3grams fat, 0grams saturated fat, 0mg cholesterol, 11.5grams carbohydrate, 3.9grams dietary fiber, 2.1grams protein.

5. CARROT PURÉE WITH OLIVE OIL AND CILANTRO

This is the perfect side dish for the holiday season, especially for patients facing pancreatic cancer, as it is a well-cooked vegetable dish which is easier to digest and less likely to aggravate digestive issues. The carrots provide an excellent source of beta-carotene. The oil may be reduced if sensitive to fat, or coconut oil may be substituted (which may be more easily absorbed). If you are sensitive to additional herbed flavors, the cilantro can be reduced or omitted. This purée can also translate well to any other root vegetable or squash – such as turnip, parsnip, acorn squash, or butternut squash.

Yield: 6 servings

INGREDIENTS:

- About 10 carrots, peeled and cubed
- 5 Tbsp. extra virgin olive oil
- Sea salt
- Fresh black pepper

- 3 Tbsp. finely chopped fresh cilantro (may substitute other fresh herbs of choice and as tolerated)

DIRECTIONS:

1. In a large pot, boil peeled and cubed carrots for about 20 minutes until they are very tender. (Alternatively, steaming them in a steam pan over boiling water may preserve the maximum amount of nutrients.)

2. In a medium pan, add fresh cilantro leaves and 3 Tbsp. of extra virgin olive oil. Heat on lowest flame for about 5 minutes.

3. Remove from heat and allow to sit for about 5 minutes.

4. Remove cilantro from oil and set aside.

5. In a food processor or using an immersion blender, add in cooked carrots and cilantro oil and 2 Tbsp. of extra virgin olive oil. Purée until smooth.

6. Add sea salt and fresh black pepper to taste and fresh cilantro as a garnish.

NUTRITIONAL DATA:

142 calories, 11.7grams fat, 1.7grams saturated fat, 0mg cholesterol, 10 grams carbohydrate, 2.5grams dietary fiber, 0.8grams protein

6. HEARTY VEGETABLE AND LENTIL SOUP

This hearty soup is very versatile and can be adapted for whatever vegetables you have available. Use this dish as a complement to a meal or serve with homemade corn bread to complete a meal. The vegetables and lentils provide an excellent amount of insoluble and soluble fiber, and this dish is a great choice for those dealing with constipation.

Yield: 6 servings

INGREDIENTS:

- 3 cups water

- 3 cups vegetable or chicken broth

- 3 medium carrots, chopped

- 1 medium onion, chopped

- 1 cup dried lentils, rinsed

- 2 celery ribs, sliced

- 1 small bell pepper, color of your choice

- 1/4 cup uncooked brown rice

- 1 bay leaf

- 1 tsp. dried basil or 1 Tbsp. of fresh chopped basil

- 1 garlic clove, minced

- 1/2 cup tomato paste

DIRECTIONS:

1. In a large saucepan, combine all ingredients except tomato paste. Bring to a boil.

2. Reduce heat; cover and simmer for 1 to 1 1/2 hours or until lentils and rice are tender.

3. Add the tomato paste and stir until blended.

4. Cook for 10-15 minutes. Discard bay leaf.

NUTRITIONAL DATA:

206 calories, 1.4grams fat, 0grams saturated fat, 0mg cholesterol, 36grams carbohydrate, 12.6grams dietary fiber, 12.9 grams protein

7. TURKEY MEATLOAF (MINI)

This healthy alternative to beef meatloaf is adaptable to those dealing with a variety of treatment-related symptoms. Providing a generous amount of protein and flavored with vegetables, this meatloaf is sure to satisfy. This is a good selection for those dealing with gastrointestinal upset like nausea or diarrhea and for those needing blander flavors and less aroma. If you are looking to spice it up, consider adding red pepper flakes or hot sauce. If looking for a lower-fat alternative, you can use turkey breast meat and add 1/4 cup more broth to this recipe for moistness.

Yield: 8 servings

INGREDIENTS:

- 1 Tbsp. olive oil

- 2 lb. ground turkey (for a leaner preference use 1 lb. breast and 1 lb. dark meat or 2 lb. breast meat for most lean option)
- 1 large or 2 small zucchini
- 2 carrots
- 1/2 medium onion
- 1 cup quick cook oats
- 3/4 cup turkey or chicken broth
- 1 Tbsp. Worcestershire sauce
- 1 Tbsp. ketchup
- 1 egg
- 1 tsp. salt
- 1 tsp. pepper

DIRECTIONS:

1. Preheat oven to 375°.

2. Shred zucchini and carrot. Slice onion finely.

3. Alternatively, you can chop ingredients in a mini food processor.

4. Sauté vegetables in olive oil on medium heat until softened, approximately 3-4 minutes.

5. While vegetables cook, add broth to oats and let soak.

6. Add cooked vegetables, oats, ketchup, Worcestershire sauce, egg, salt, and pepper to ground turkey.

5. Mix ingredients together, avoid overmixing.

7. Place mixture in a meatloaf shape in a rectangular baking dish and bake for 1 hour and internal thermometer reads at least 165°.

8. For extra crispy top, broil for the last 5 minutes of cooking, watching closely to avoid burning.

TIP: you can also make "mini meatloafs" in a muffin pan or miniature loaf pans, or even on a sheet pan shaped into 8 smaller loafs. These are great for freezing and lend themselves well to a leftover meatloaf sandwich.

NUTRITIONAL DATA:
324 calories, 16.3grams fat, 2.8grams saturated fat, 146mg cholesterol, 11.6grams carbohydrate, 2grams dietary fiber, 37.8 grams protein

8. SWEET POTATO AND WHITE BEAN FRITTERS

Trying this unique plant-based recipe will add vibrancy and texture to your plate. Substitute any squash or beans that you have available. This recipe is a good choice for those needing foods that are soft and easy to chew and swallow.

Yield: 12 fritters

INGREDIENTS:

- 2 cups (10 oz.) cubed and peeled sweet potato
- 1 can (15.5 oz.) no-added salt white beans, drained and rinsed
- 4 Tbsp. quick cooking oats

40

- 1 large egg

- 1/4 cup onion, minced

- 1 large clove garlic, minced

- 2 tsp. chopped fresh sage leaves

- 1/4 tsp. cumin

- Salt and freshly ground pepper to taste

- 1 Tbsp. canola oil or extra virgin olive oil, divided

- 3/4 cup low-fat sour cream or fat-free plain Greek-style yogurt

DIRECTIONS:

1. In large saucepan with a steamer basket, steam sweet potatoes until tender, about 15-17 minutes.

2. Transfer sweet potato to food processor. Add beans, oats, egg, onion, garlic, sage, cumin. Pulse until blended yet slightly chunky.

3. Season with salt and pepper.

4. Heat 1 Tbsp. oil in large skillet over medium-high heat.

5. Gently drop six 1/4 cup portions of mixture into pan and gently press into round patties with back of measuring cup or spatula. Don't over crowd skillet.

6. Sauté fritters until golden brown on bottom, about 5 minutes. Heat may need to be adjusted for optimal browning.

7. Carefully turn over each fritter and sauté until other side is golden brown, about 3-4 minutes.

6. Transfer fritters to plate and cover with foil to keep warm.

7. Use remaining oil to sauté remaining six fritters. There should be 12 fritters in total.

8. Serve warm with sour cream or Greek yogurt.

NUTRITIONAL DATA:

104 calories, 4.9grams fat, 2.1grams saturated fat, 22mg cholesterol, 12.5grams carbohydrate, 2.7grams dietary fiber, 3.7grams protein

9. RICE PUDDING

A creamy, often well-tolerated, high-calorie pudding that works as a great dessert for those needing to add protein and calories to their daily intake. For those requiring a lower fat alternative, reduced-fat milk may be substituted. Non-dairy, lactose-free options like soy, rice, or almond milk can work as well.

Yield: 4 servings

INGREDIENTS:

- 2 cups of whole milk, reduced-fat milk, or non-dairy alternative
- 1/3 cup of sugar
- 3/4 cups of long grain white or brown rice

44

- 1/4 tsp. salt

- 1 egg (beaten)

- 1/2 tsp. vanilla extract

- 1/4 cup dried fruit of your choice (optional)

- Cinnamon or nutmeg for sprinkling on top (optional)

DIRECTIONS:

1. First rinse uncooked rice with cold water.

2. Bring 1 1/2 cups of water to a boil.

3. Add rice, reduce heat, and cook for approximately 20 minutes until tender.

4. In large pot add rice, 1 1/2 cups milk, sugar and salt.

5. Stir rice constantly to avoid rice from sticking to bottom of pot.

6. Cook until mixture is a thick and creamy texture, approximately 20 minutes.

7. Remove pot from heat, and while still hot, add remaining 1/2 cup milk, beaten eggs (add very slowly while stirring pot), vanilla, and optional dried fruit (such as raisins).

8. Return to medium heat and stir again until slightly thickened (5-10 minutes max).

9. Remove from heat, and pour into containers. Top with a sprinkling of cinnamon or nutmeg for garnish as desired.

10. Refrigerate before serving.

Tip: for extra cinnamon flavor, boil rice with a cinnamon stick added to the water

NUTRITIONAL DATA:

289 calories, 5.9grams fat, 0.5grams saturated fat, 59mg cholesterol, 50grams carbohydrate, 1.2grams dietary fiber, 8.1grams protein

10. BANANA BLUEBERRY MUFFINS

These muffins are a great quick breakfast treat, with bananas and blueberries providing soluble fiber, potassium, and phytonutrients. Non-dairy milk can be substituted for those who are intolerant to lactose and whole-wheat flour can be substituted to increase the fiber content.

Yield: 12 muffins

INGREDIENTS:

- 1/2 cup mashed ripe banana (about 1 large)
- 1/2 cup granulated sugar
- 1/2 cup milk (may also sub any non-dairy milk)
- 1/3 cup canola oil
- 1 Tbsp. vanilla extract
- 1 tsp. cinnamon
- 1 cup all-purpose flour (or whole wheat flour)
- 2 tsp. baking powder

- 1/2 cup frozen blueberries

DIRECTIONS:

1. Preheat oven to 400°.

2. Line muffin pan with paper cups.

3. In a large bowl, mash the banana with a fork.

4. Add the sugar, milk, oil, vanilla, cinnamon, and whisk until combined.

5. Add the flour, baking powder, and stir until just combined; don't over mix.

6. Fold in 1/2 cup frozen blueberries.

7. Add batter to muffin tin (for easy distribution use medium cookie scoop)

8. Bake for 15-20 minutes, or until tops are slightly golden

NUTRITIONAL DATA:

125 calories, 6.4grams fat, 0.6grams saturated fat, 1mg cholesterol, 15.5grams carbohydrate, 0.7grams dietary fiber, 1.5grams protein

11. BAKED BERRY FRENCH TOAST

This French toast recipe is great to make ahead of time for a busy weekday morning. It is a good balanced entrée that includes protein, carbohydrates, dairy, and fruit. Cream cheese and milk components can be substituted with lactose-free versions for those experiencing lactose intolerance.

Yield: 8 Servings

INGREDIENTS:

- 12 slices day-old bread, cut into
- 1-inch cubes
- 1 (12 oz.) package of low-fat cream cheese, room temperature
- 2 1/4 cups low-fat fat-free milk or non-dairy alternative, divided
- 2 tsp. vanilla, divided
- 2 cups blueberries, fresh or thawed frozen, divided
- 10 eggs, beaten
- 1/4 cup plus 1 Tbsp. honey or pure maple syrup

DIRECTIONS:
1. Preheat oven to 350°.

51

2. Lightly grease a 9x13 inch-baking dish.

3. Blend 1 brick of cream cheese, 1/4 cup of milk, 1 Tbsp. honey and 1 tsp. vanilla.

4. Arrange 1/2 of the bread cubes in bottom of dish. Top with cream cheese mixture. Sprinkle 1 cup of blueberries over top, and top with remaining bread cubes.

5. In large bowl, mix eggs, milk, vanilla extract, and honey or syrup. Pour over bread cubes and Cover, refrigerate for 1 hour or overnight.

6. Cover, and bake for 30 minutes. Uncover, and continue baking for 25-30 minutes, until center is firm and surface is lightly browned.

7. Let cool for 10-12 minutes. Top with remaining berries and enjoy.

NUTRITIONAL DATA:

231 calories, 7.5grams fat, 1.7grams saturated fat, 205mg cholesterol, 29grams carbohydrate, 3.8grams dietary fiber, 13.7grams protein

12. PUMPKIN OATMEAL BARS

These are a healthy alternative to many common cookie recipes. Whole-wheat flour, oats, pumpkin, and ground flaxseed add soluble and insoluble fiber, along with the phytochemical and antioxidant benefits of the added spices. Great selections for an after dinner dessert or midday snack. Flaxseed can be omitted if experiencing gas, bloating, or diarrhea.

Yield: 40 square bars or 48 cookies

INGREDIENTS:

- 2 cups whole-wheat flour
- 1 1/3 cups rolled oats
- 1 tsp. baking soda
- 3/4 tsp. salt
- 1 tsp. cinnamon
- 1/2 tsp. nutmeg
- 1 1/3 cup sugar
- 2/3 cup canola oil
- 3 Tbsp. molasses

- 1 can of cooked pumpkin puree

- 1 tsp. vanilla

- 2 Tbsp. ground flaxseed (optional)

- Optional add-ins: 1 cup mini chocolate chips

DIRECTIONS:

1. Preheat oven to 350°. Grease two 12 x 17 baking sheet pans.

2. Mix together flour, oats, baking soda, salt, and spices.

3. In a separate bowl, mix together sugar, oil, molasses, pumpkin, vanilla, and optional flaxseeds until very well combined.

4. Mix flour and sugar mixtures together. Fold in chocolate chips, if desired.

5. Spread and press batter onto greased cookie sheets (to make cookies, drop 1 inch size balls of batter an inch apart, and flatten tops of cookies with fork or your fingers to press into cookie shape).

6. Bake for 16 minutes or until inserted knife

7. or toothpick is clean. Rotate halfway

8. through baking.

9. Remove from oven (if making cookies, transfer to wire rack to cool).

10. Once cool slice into 20 bars per sheet pan.

NUTRITIONAL DATA:

101 calories, 4grams fat, 0grams saturated fat, 0mg cholesterol, 15.4grams carbohydrate, 0.9grams dietary fiber, 1.2grams protein

13. ASPARAGUS FRITTATA

Frittatas are very versatile – they can be used at any meal as a main dish, side dish or appetizer, and can easily be turned into a quiche by adding a pie crust at the bottom (if able to tolerate higher amounts of fat). Eggs provide the highest quality protein available in any food. This recipe is great for those needing easy to chew/swallowing foods.

Yield: 1 9-inch quiche, serves 6

INGREDIENTS:

- ½ lb. fresh asparagus, trimmed and cut into ½ inch pieces
- 1 egg white, lightly beaten

- 4 eggs, beaten

- 1 ½ cups fat-free or low-fat milk

- 1/4 tsp. ground nutmeg

- 1 Tbsp. Dijon mustard

- 1 cup shredded Swiss or muenster cheese (use reduced fat cheese if experiencing fat intolerance)

- Salt and pepper to taste

DIRECTIONS:

1. Preheat oven to 375°.

2. Add asparagus to saucepan with 1 inch of water or place in a steamer. Steam for 4-6 minutes or until tender but not mushy. Once steamed, allow it to drain well and cool.

3. Coat pie dish with nonstick cooking spray.

4. Add drained and dried asparagus to pie dish.

5. In a bowl, beat together eggs, milk, mustard, nutmeg, salt and pepper. Add shredded cheese and mix in.

6. Pour egg mixture into pie pan.

7. Bake uncovered in preheated oven until firm, about 40-50 minutes.

8. Enjoy warm or at room temperature.

NUTRITIONAL DATA:

125 calories, 8.8 grams fat, 4.6 grams saturated fat, 127 mg cholesterol, 2.2 grams carbohydrate, 0.9 grams dietary fiber, 9.9 grams protein

14. VEGETABLE POPOVER

These vegetable popovers are excellent for individuals needing soft, easy-to-swallow foods. Eggs (or egg substitute) add an excellent source of high-quality protein. This is also a great recipe to prepare ahead of time and reheat as a healthy mini-meal.

Yield: 6 servings

INGREDIENTS:

- 1 zucchini, chopped into bite-size pieces
- 1 large carrot, chopped into small pieces (about half the size of the zucchini)
- 2 tsp. olive oil

- 6 large eggs

- 1/4 cup milk (non-dairy alternative, if desired)

- 1/3 cup shredded cheddar cheese (use reduced-fat cheese for those experiencing fat intolerance)

- Salt and freshly ground black pepper, to taste

- Pinch of turmeric

- Onion powder, to taste

DIRECTIONS:

1. Preheat the oven to 350°.

1. Spray 6 muffin cups with nonstick spray.

2. Sauté the zucchini and the carrots in 2 tsp. olive oil for 5-7 minutes.

3. In a medium bowl, whisk together the eggs and milk. Add salt, pepper, turmeric, and onion powder.

4. Distribute egg mixture evenly into muffin cups.

5. Distribute zucchini and carrots into egg mixture.

6. Bake 25 to 30 minutes, or until egg is cooked through.

NUTRITIONAL DATA:

126 calories, 8.9 grams fat, 3.2grams saturated fat, 193 mg cholesterol, 3.4 grams carbohydrate, 0.7 grams dietary fiber, 8.7grams protein

15. CHICKEN WITH QUINOA

This recipe has "pack a protein punch", but for additional protein add white beans and cook the quinoa in chicken broth. To add additional flavor or variety, top with low-fat sour cream and salsa for a Mexican-inspired dish. Other grains such as bulgur, rice, or couscous can also be used.

Yield: 6 servings

INGREDIENTS:

- 1 Tbsp. olive oil, divided
- 1 lb. ground chicken breast
- 1 tsp. rosemary
- Pinch salt (optional)
- 1/4 tsp. pepper (optional)

- 1 cup quinoa

- 1 1/2 cups frozen kale

- 1/4 cup chicken broth

DIRECTIONS:

1. Heat 2 tsp. olive oil in skillet; add the ground chicken, rosemary, salt, and pepper.

2. Cook until cooked through and browned.

3. Add frozen kale and chicken broth and allow to thaw and wilt; approximately 2-3 minutes.

4. While the chicken is cooking, separately cook quinoa according to package directions in medium size saucepan with remaining tsp. of olive oil. Fluff with fork when cooked.

5. Add quinoa to skillet with chicken and kale and combine well. Serve warm.

These recipes were developed by registered dietitians who are board-certified specialists in oncology nutrition

NUTRITIONAL DATA:
217 calories, 4.8 grams fat, 0.6 grams saturated fat, 47 mg cholesterol, 19.9 grams carbohydrate, 2.8 grams dietary fiber, 23.9 grams protein

16. CHICKEN KEBAB WITH TZATZIKI AND PITA

A great summer time chicken recipe topped with cool, creamy tzatziki sauce. Preparation is required

2-3 hours ahead of time but well worth the extra wait time. Choose this recipe for those needing high protein, low fiber choices.

Yield: 6 servings

INGREDIENTS:

Pita:

- 1 pack store-bought pita bread

- Tzatziki sauce:

- 3 cucumbers

- 12 oz. plain Greek yogurt

- 1 pinch of sea salt

- 1/2 tsp. extra virgin olive oil

- 2 cloves of garlic, minced

Chicken:

- 1 ½ pounds skinless, boneless chicken breast halves, cut into 1/2 inch pieces

- 1/4 cup olive oil for marinade

- 2 Tbsp. lemon juice

- 1 tsp. dried oregano

- ½ tsp. sea salt

- 6 wooden skewers

NUTRITIONAL DATA:

441 calories, 13.8 grams fat, 3 grams saturated fat, 67 mg cholesterol, 44.7 grams carbohydrate, 3 grams dietary fiber, 34.9 grams protein

DIRECTIONS:

Tzatziki sauce:

1. Clean and grate cucumbers. Be sure to remove seeds and peel off cucumber skin if on a low-fiber diet.

2. Strain juice and place in medium bowl.

3. Add yogurt to bowl and mix cucumbers, garlic, salt and olive oil together.

4. Cover and refrigerate for 30 minutes.

Chicken and pita:

1. Combine 1/4 cup olive oil, lemon juice, 1 tsp. oregano, and 1/2 tsp. sea salt in a large bowl.

2. Add chicken, mix with the marinade and cover the bowl.

3. Marinate in the refrigerator for at least 2 hours.

4. Skewer chicken evenly on 6 wooden skewers.

5. Preheat grill, place pitas on grill for 2 minutes on each side until slightly browned.

6. Remove from grill and set aside.

7. Cook the skewers on the preheated grill, turning frequently until nicely browned on all sides, about 10 minutes per side.

8. Serve with grilled pita and topped with tzatziki sauce.

17. EDAMAME HUMMUS WRAP

Soy is a high-quality protein that does not cause the same discomfort that other beans and hummuses can. This recipe is extremely easy and satisfying. Can be delicious plain or with any added vegetables that you can tolerate (those with diarrhea or indigestion should be sure to use well-cooked vegetables without the skin).

Yield: 4 servings

INGREDIENTS:

- 1 cup cooked shelled edamame
- 1/4 cup Tahini (sesame paste)
- 1 Tbsp. lemon juice

- Garlic clove, peeled

- 2 Tbsp. coarsely chopped fresh herbs (such as rosemary, thyme, and basil)

- 2 Tbsp. olive oil

- Salt to taste (approximately 1/4 tsp.)

- 4 flour wraps

- Optional: Sautéed or roasted vegetables, or fresh, raw vegetables that you can tolerate

DIRECTIONS:

1. Combine edamame, tahini, lemon juice, garlic,

2. and herbs in food processor.

3. Process ingredients until smooth.

4. Drizzle olive oil through feed tube of food processor, continuing to process until the oil

is fully incorporated into the hummus mixture.

5. Season with salt to taste.

6. Spread 1/4 cup hummus in each wrap, top with raw or roasted vegetables of choice, roll and serve.

NUTRITIONAL DATA:

399 calories, 21.9 grams fat, 3.1 grams saturated fat, 0 mg cholesterol, 39.9 grams carbohydrate, 4.1grams dietary fiber, 12.1 grams protein

18. CHICKEN SALAD SANDWICH

This sandwich is very easy to prepare and contains satisfying flavors and textures. It is a well-balanced meal that includes protein and carbohydrates, along with a splash of colorful fruit and herbs. For those experiencing fat intolerance, reduced fat mayo can be substituted and walnuts can be avoided. You can also experiment with other herbs like rosemary or basil for varied flavors.

Yield: 4 sandwiches

INGREDIENTS:

- 2 chicken breasts (skin on during cooking only) or approximately

- 2 cups diced or shredded cooked, skinless chicken

- 2 Tbsp. mayonnaise (may substitute yogurt - low fat or Greek - and 1 tsp. lemon juice)

- 1/4 cup sliced grapes

- 2 Tbsp. dried cranberries

- 1/4 cup chopped walnuts (optional)

- 2 tsp. dried tarragon

- 8 slices bread

DIRECTIONS:

1. Preheat oven to 375°.

2. Roast chicken breasts for approximately 45 minutes until cooked through, juices run clear and temperature of chicken reaches 165°.

3. Remove skin from breast meat. Discard skin. Cube, dice, or shred meat.

4. Add mayonnaise, grapes, cranberries, walnuts, and tarragon.

5. Mix well and divide into 4 (~3/4 cup) portions and spread onto bread.

Delicious with toasted bread

NUTRITIONAL DATA:
237 calories, 9.8 grams fat, 1.4 grams saturated fat, 56 mg cholesterol, 13.1 grams carbohydrate, 1.2 grams dietary fiber, 23.7 grams protein

19. SUMMER VEGETABLES OMELET

This omelet is an excellent source of protein and includes squash, which is generally a well-tolerated vegetable. Cheddar cheese can be substituted for another flavor of cheese, or lactose free cheese for those who are lactose intolerant.

Yield: Two 2-egg omelets

INGREDIENTS:

- 2/3 cup sliced summer squash

- 2/3 cup sliced fresh zucchini

- 2 Tbsp. oil, divided

- 4 eggs, beaten, divided (may substitute

2 egg whites for each egg if needed for

lower fat intake)

• 2 slices white cheddar cheese (use

reduced fat cheese if experiencing

fat intolerance or any flavor cheese

of choice)

DIRECTIONS:
1. Heat 1 Tbsp. oil in omelet pan over medium heat.
2. Sauté zucchini and squash in oil for 4-5 minutes until tender.
3. Remove vegetables and keep warm.

4. Add additional Tbsp. oil to warm pan. Add two beaten eggs and half of the vegetables.

5. Flip and cook thoroughly. Fold in half and top with 1 slice of white cheddar cheese.

6. Make second omelet with remaining ingredients.

NUTRITIONAL DATA:

310 calories, 27.4 grams fat, 9.1 grams saturated fat, 193 mg cholesterol, 3.6 grams carbohydrate, 0.8 grams dietary fiber, 13.4 grams protein

20. SHRIMP POMODORO & ANGEL HAIR

This delicious shrimp dish provides a great source of protein, but can be substituted for chicken for those who may be allergic to shellfish. Tomato content can be reduced to a smaller quantity of diced tomato or omitted and replaced with chicken or vegetable broth in order to reduce acid content. In addition, herbs and spices can be adapted to suit flavor preferences and digestive tolerance. For those looking to add more dietary fiber, whole wheat pasta can be substituted. For those who are experiencing fat malabsorption or dairy intolerance, olive oil can be reduced and parmigiano cheese can be omitted.

Yield: 6 Servings

INGREDIENTS:

- 1 lb. angel hair pasta
- 6 Tbsp. extra virgin olive oil
- 3 sprigs fresh thyme
- 8 cloves garlic (sliced paper thin)
- 3/4 cup finely chopped onion
- 1 cup tomato concasse (peeled, seeds removed, diced)
- 1 Tbsp. tomato paste
- 1/2 cup non-alcoholic cooking wine
- 2 Tbsp. chiffonade fresh basil (stacked basil leaves, tightly rolled, thinly sliced)
- 3 Tbsp. crushed red pepper flakes** (optional)
- 1 1/2 lb. size 16/20 wild shrimp

- Kosher salt (as needed)

- Fresh ground pepper (as needed)

- 1 Tbsp. minced Italian parsley

- 4 Tbsp. parmigiano cheese (optional)

DIRECTIONS FOR SAUCE:

1. In a medium sized sauce pan add 3 Tbsp. of extra virgin olive oil over medium heat and add onions. Sweat onions for 5 minutes until translucent, then add half the amount of garlic, red

1. pepper flakes (if wanted), 2 sprigs of thyme and tomato paste.

2. Continue to cook over medium heat for 3 minutes. Add white wine (reserving 1 Tbsp. for shrimp).

3. Continue to stir and cook until wine is evaporated. Add tomato concasse, 1 tsp. kosher salt and desired amount of fresh ground pepper. Lower heat to slow simmer for 45 minutes.

4. After 45 minutes, with a hand blender, pulse to slightly puree (you do not want the sauce to be completely smooth). Pulses should be 15 2-second pulses.

5. Add parsley. Reserve for plating.

DIRECTIONS FOR SHRIMP:

1. In a medium sauté pan that's been pre-heated over medium-high heat, add the remaining olive oil and garlic.

2. When the garlic begins to slightly brown, add shrimp that has been shelled and de-veined, season with salt and pepper. Sauté for 1-2 minutes over high heat.

3. Add remaining fresh thyme and 1 Tbsp of white wine. Remove from heat.

4. Reserve for plate assembly.

DIRECTIONS FOR PASTA:

1. In a large stock pot add 2 gallons of water and 3 Tbsp. kosher salt; bring to a boil.

2. Add angel hair pasta and boil for 3 minutes, achieving doneness of al dente.

3. Strain pasta and put pasta back into pot.

4. Add 3/4 cup tomato sauce to coat pasta.

METHOD FOR ASSEMBLY:

1. Heat shrimp in remaining tomato sauce. Place desired amount of pasta into a pasta bowl.

2. Spoon over tomato sauce. Add desired amount of shrimp and fresh basil. Each dish can be garnished with 1 Tbsp. parmigiano cheese

NUTRITIONAL DATA:

497 calories, 17.8 grams fat, 3.4 grams saturated fat, 189 mg cholesterol, 49.3 grams carbohydrate, 1.8 grams dietary fiber, 34 grams protein

21. SALMON BURGER WITH BOK CHOY, GINGER AND LEMONGRASS

Salmon burgers provide a tasty alternative to old-fashioned beef burgers along with the benefit of healthy omega-3 fats. These burgers have a refreshing appeal from the lemongrass and ginger. Top with traditional plant-based burger topping on a hearty whole-grain roll. Tuna can be substituted for salmon as well. For those sensitive to spices, they can be toned down as needed.

Yield: 4 Servings

INGREDIENTS:

- 1 lb. salmon fillet (or canned salmon)

- 3 cups bok choy, chopped finely (green leafy top only)
- 3 scallions, minced
- 1 Tbsp. finely grated ginger (peeled)
- 1 Tbsp. finely grated lemongrass (dried lemongrass can be substituted if fresh is not found)
- Salt and pepper to taste
- 1 large egg white
- 1 Tbsp. soy sauce
- Cilantro (optional)

DIRECTIONS:

1. Cut salmon into 1/4 inch dice (or use canned salmon), stir into mixture of bok choy,

scallions, ginger, lemongrass, salt and pepper in large bowl until combined.

2. Beat together egg white and soy sauce in a small bowl and stir into salmon mixture.

3. Form into four patties that are 1/2 inch thick.

4. Heat non-stick skillet over medium heat. Add 1 Tbsp. of olive oil to cover bottom of skillet.

5. Add salmon patties, cooking for approximately 3-4 minutes per side.

6. Serve hot.

7. Top with cilantro leaves, if desired.

NUTRITIONAL DATA:

173 calories, 7.2 grams fat, 1 gram saturated fat, 50 mg cholesterol, 3.6 grams carbohydrate, 1 gram dietary fiber, 24.3 grams protein

22. PEACHES AND CREAM SMOOTHIE

Simple meals like shakes and smoothies are often helpful ways for people caring for or living with pancreatic cancer to get the nutrients they need. This Peaches and Cream Smoothie combines the potassium and fiber benefits of peaches and bananas along with soluble fiber from rolled oats, which can help to alleviate loose bowel movements and promote regularity. The protein powder can be added at the recommendation of your healthcare team for additional nutritional value. Dairy components can be easily substituted with lactose-free or non-dairy versions.

Yield: 1-2 servings

INGREDIENTS:

- ½ cup rolled oats

- cup plain yogurt (or soy/coconut/almond yogurt)

- ¾ cup milk (or soy/almond/rice milk) + ¼ cup more for morning

- 1 small ripe peach (or ½ cup frozen peaches, thawed and softened)

- ½ medium banana

- Pinch of salt

- 1-2 Tbsp. protein powder (whey or soy) (optional)

DIRECTIONS:

1. Gather all ingredients

2. Combine ingredients in a blender, blend until smooth

3. Store in a container in your refrigerator overnight if making ahead of time. In the morning, add last ¼ cup milk, more if you need it to blend smoothly.

Nutritional Data:

(assumes regular whole milk and yogurt)

426 calories, 9 grams fat, 4.5 grams saturated fat, 25 mg cholesterol, 68 grams carbohydrate, 7grams dietary fiber, 20 grams protein

23. TURKEY SWEET POTATO HASH

Since fatigue is sometimes experienced by people living with pancreatic cancer, this easy-to-prepare dish is nutrient dense and a good source of protein and B vitamins, which can help boost energy. In addition, the cooked apple and sweet potato provide fiber that is easily tolerated and full of antioxidants like beta-carotene and quercetin. The ingredients include a variety of appealing textures and flavors of the holiday season.

Yield: 6 servings, 1 ¼ cups each

INGREDIENTS
- 2 medium sweet potatoes, peeled and cut into ½-inch pieces

91

- 1 medium apple, cored and cut into ½-inch pieces (Honeycrisp or Braeburn work wonderfully, although any apple can suit this recipe)
- ½ cup reduced-fat sour cream (may also substitute reduced-fat yogurt)
- 1 tsp. lemon juice
- 1 Tbsp. olive oil
- 1 medium shallot, chopped
- 3 cups diced, cooked, skinless turkey breast (or chicken)
- 1 tsp. dried rosemary (1 Tbsp. fresh, chopped)
- Salt and pepper, to taste

DIRECTIONS:

1. Place sweet potatoes in a steamer basket and cook for approximately 10 minutes.

2. Add apple and cook until everything is just tender, about 3 minutes longer.

3. Be sure that they are not overly mushy. Drain and set aside.

4. Transfer 1 cup of the mixture to a large bowl; mash. Stir in sour cream and lemon juice.

5. Add the remaining sweet potato/apple mixture and stir gently to mix.

6. Heat oil in a large skillet over medium-high heat. Add shallot until softened, 1 to 2

minutes. Add turkey (or chicken), rosemary, salt and pepper.

7. Stir mixture occasionally and cook until heated through, about 2 minutes.

8. Add the reserved sweet potato apple mixture to the pan. Press on the hash with a wide metal spoon or spatula. Cook hash until the bottom is lightly browned, about 3 minutes.

9. Divide into multiple sections with spatula; flip and cook until the bottom sides are browned, about 2 to 3 minutes.

10. Serve promptly

Nutritional Data:

174 calories, 6 grams fat, 2 grams saturated fat, 38 mg cholesterol, 17 grams carbohydrate, 2grams dietary fiber, 14 grams protein.

24. TURKEY TORTELLINI SOUP

Many people with pancreatic cancer often will better tolerate and enjoy simple, comforting meals. This classic soup recipe can be the base for a warm and hearty soup.

Yield: 8 Servings

INGREDIENTS

- One 12-15 lb. turkey

- 3 medium-size onions

- 6 garlic cloves

- 6 large carrots

- 1 head of celery

- 3 bay leaves

- 6 sprigs fresh thyme

- 1 sprig rosemary

- 3 cups cheese tortellini

- 1 bunch parsley

- ½ cup parmigiano cheese

- ¼ cup extra virgin olive oil

DIRECTIONS:

For Roasting the Turkey

1. Preheat oven to 350°.

2. Place turkey on roasting rack. Season inside and out with salt and pepper.

3. Roast turkey for 2 ½ or 3 hours until internal temperature reaches 155°, basting with natural juices every 30 minutes.

4. Remove turkey and lightly dome with aluminum foil.

1. Allow to cool. Once cool, remove skin and debone turkey.

5. Place body and all bones back into the roasting pan. Roast at 350° for 30 minutes, until bones are dark, golden brown.

6. Shred turkey meat into bite size pieces.

7. Reserve.

For the Turkey Stock

1. In a large stock pot, place turkey bones and body, ½ head of celery (chopped), 3 carrots (chopped), 2 onions (chopped), 4 garlic cloves (smashed), 3 bay leaves, 1 sprig rosemary and 6 sprigs thyme.

2. Cover with 4 inches of water, bring to a simmer.

3. Lower heat and slowly simmer stock for 2 hours, occasionally skimming fat from the top.

4. After 2 hours, strain stock through a fine sift and cheese cloth.

5. Cool and reserve.

For the Garnish

1. Remaining celery, small dice (quarter by quarter inch)

2. Remaining carrots, small dice (quarter by quarter inch)

3. Remaining onions, small dice (quarter by quarter inch)

4. Remaining garlic, minced

5. In a large stock pot, put 2 gallons of water. Add 2 Tbsp. of kosher salt. Bring to a rolling boil and add the tortellini.

6. Cook for 6 minutes, occasionally stirring. Strain.

7. Toss 1 Tbsp. extra virgin olive oil into the tortellini.

8. Lay flat on a sheet tray and allow to cool in refrigerator.

9. Reserve.

To Assemble the Soup

1. Add stock to large stock pot.

2. Add all diced vegetables and bring to a simmer. Cook until carrots are tender, approximately 6-8 minutes.

3. Add shredded turkey meat, tortellini, and finely chopped parsley. Adjust soup seasoning with desired amount of kosher salt and fresh ground pepper.

To Serve

1. In a soup bowl, place 1 large ladle of garnish into center of bowl, top the bowl off with stock.

2. Drizzle with ½ tsp. extra virgin olive oil over the top of the soup.

3. Add 1 Tbsp. of grated parmigiano cheese

Nutritional Data: (assumes 1 oz turkey per bowl)
338 calories, 13 grams fat, 3 grams saturated fat, 39mg cholesterol, 37grams carbohydrate, 2.5grams dietary fiber, 19 grams protein.

FINAL THOUGHT

Pancreatitis can be a painful and frustrating condition, especially when it becomes chronic. There isn't a single pancreatitis diet that works for everyone, but diet can have a big impact on how you feel. Know that finding the right plan for you can take time, and work with your doctor, a registered dietician, and/or nutritionist to fine-tune a pancreatic diet that meets your needs.

Nutrition plays a vital role in treating pancreatitis. The impact of this disease in patients can be devastating if left unmanaged. Once a patient has been diagnosed with pancreatitis, proper diet and nutrition is the main goal for pancreatitis management to help with the impact of the disease in the patient. These specific goals are crucial in the treatment and management of the disease.

The content in this book is not intended to be a substitute for professional medical advice, diagnosis or treatment. Talk to your healthcare team for nutritional advice or specific questions you have about managing your condition or that of a loved one.

Printed in the USA
CPSIA information can be obtained
at www.ICGtesting.com
CBHW070904301124
18254CB00035B/900